FAITH
A BIBLE VERSE PICTURE BOOK

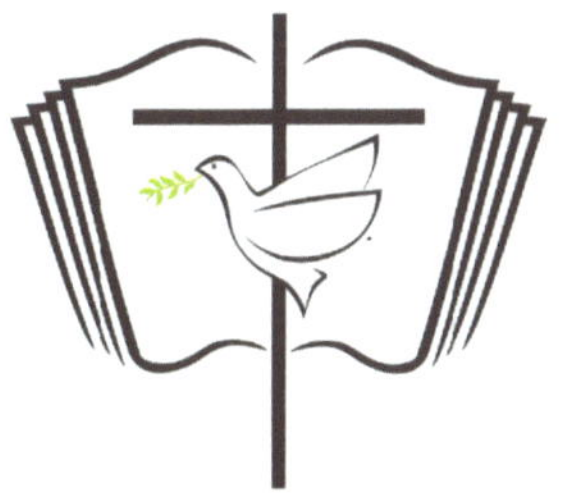

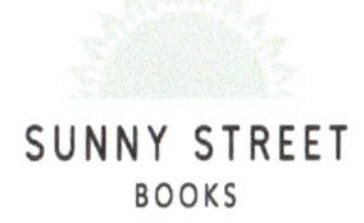

SUNNY STREET
BOOKS

Mark 11:24

Therefore I tell you,
whatever you ask for in
prayer, believe that you
have received it, and it
will be yours.

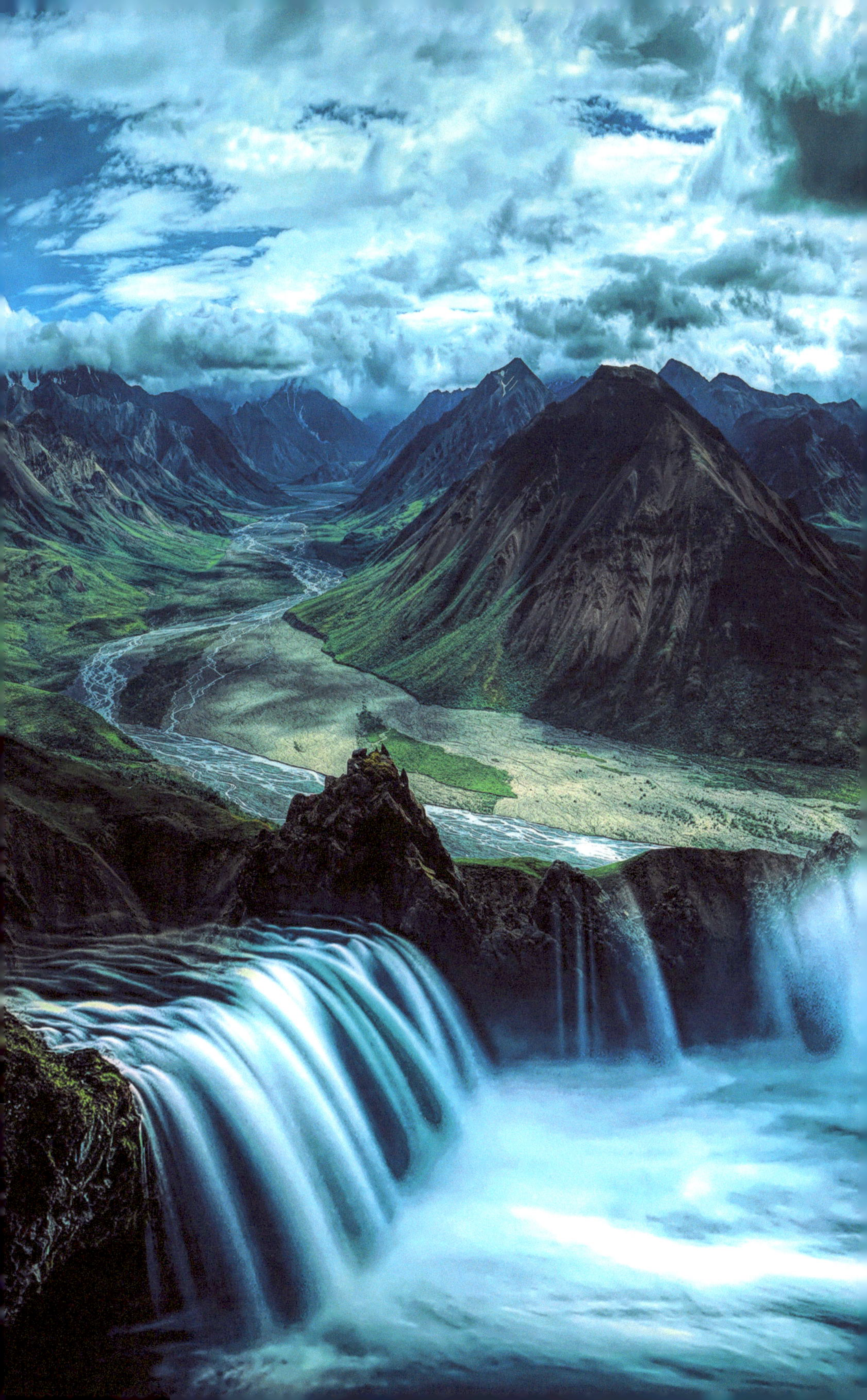

Matthew 17-20

Truly I tell you, if you have faith as small as a mustard seed, you can say to this mountain, "Move from here to there," and it will move. Nothing will be impossible for you.

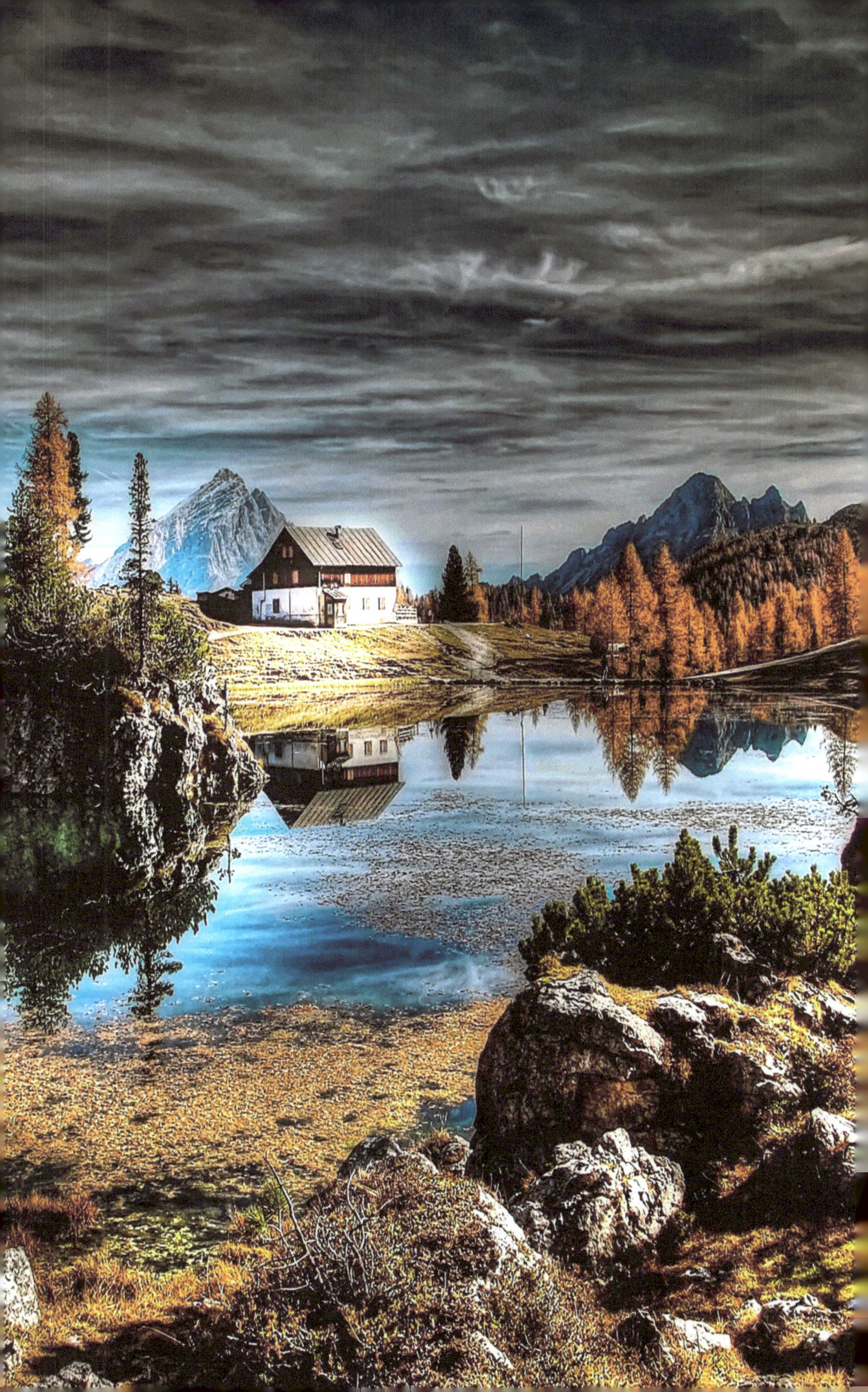

2 Timothy 4-7

I have fought the good fight,

I have finished the race,

I have kept the faith.

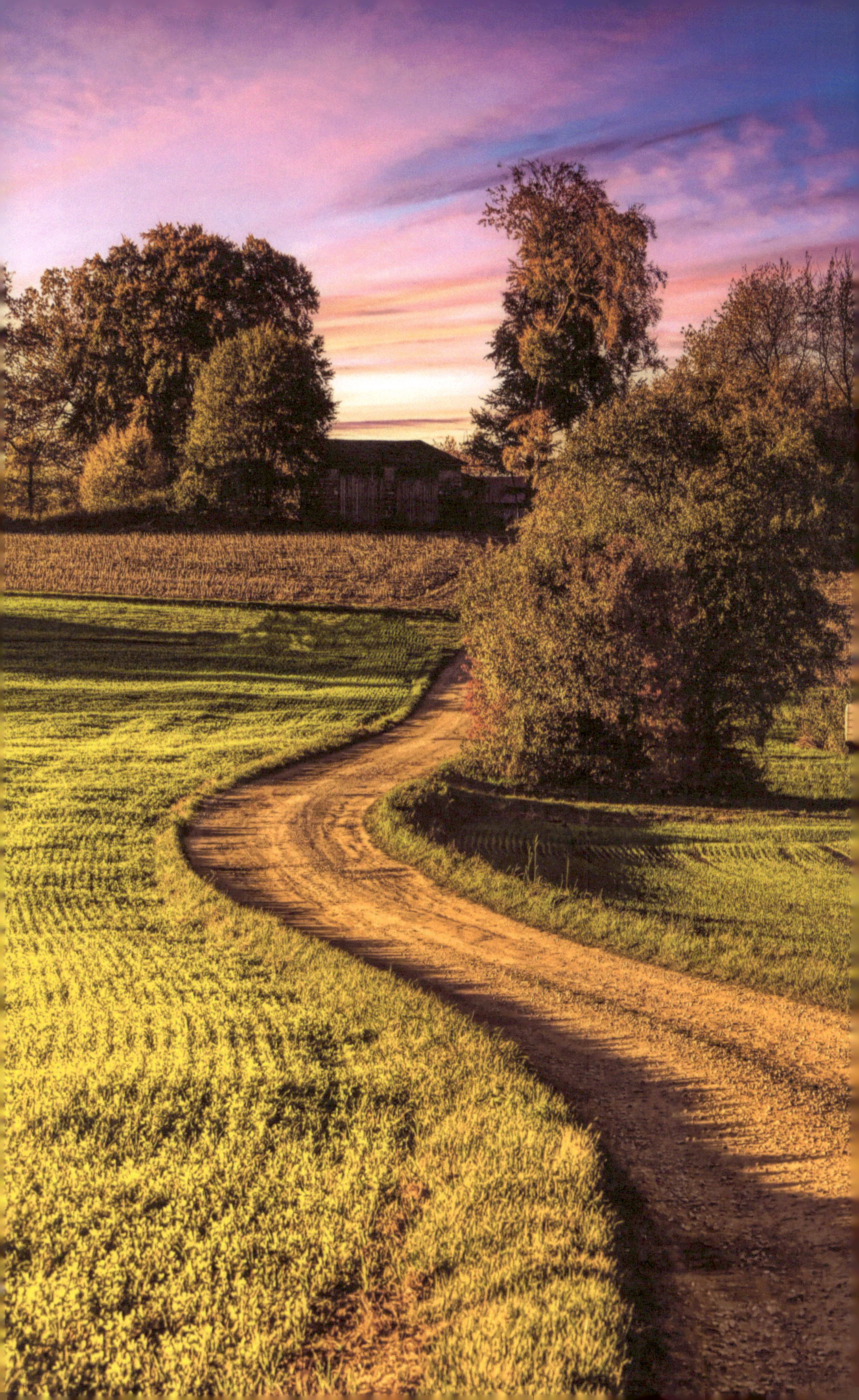

Hebrews 11:1

Now faith is confidence

in what we hope for and

assurance about what we

do not see.

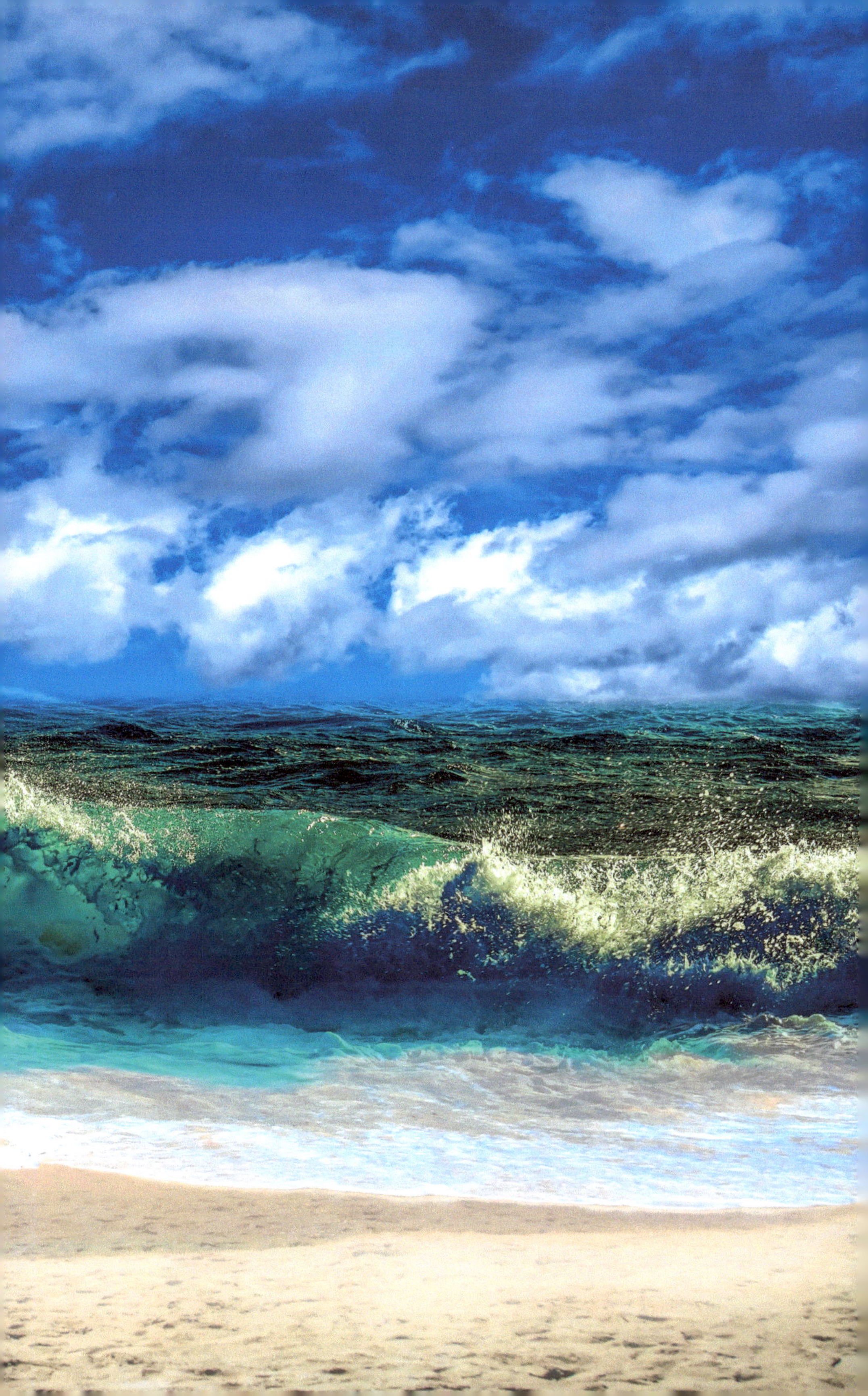

Matthew 15-28

Then Jesus said to her,
"O woman, your faith is
great; it shall be done
for you as you wish."
And her daughter was
healed at once.

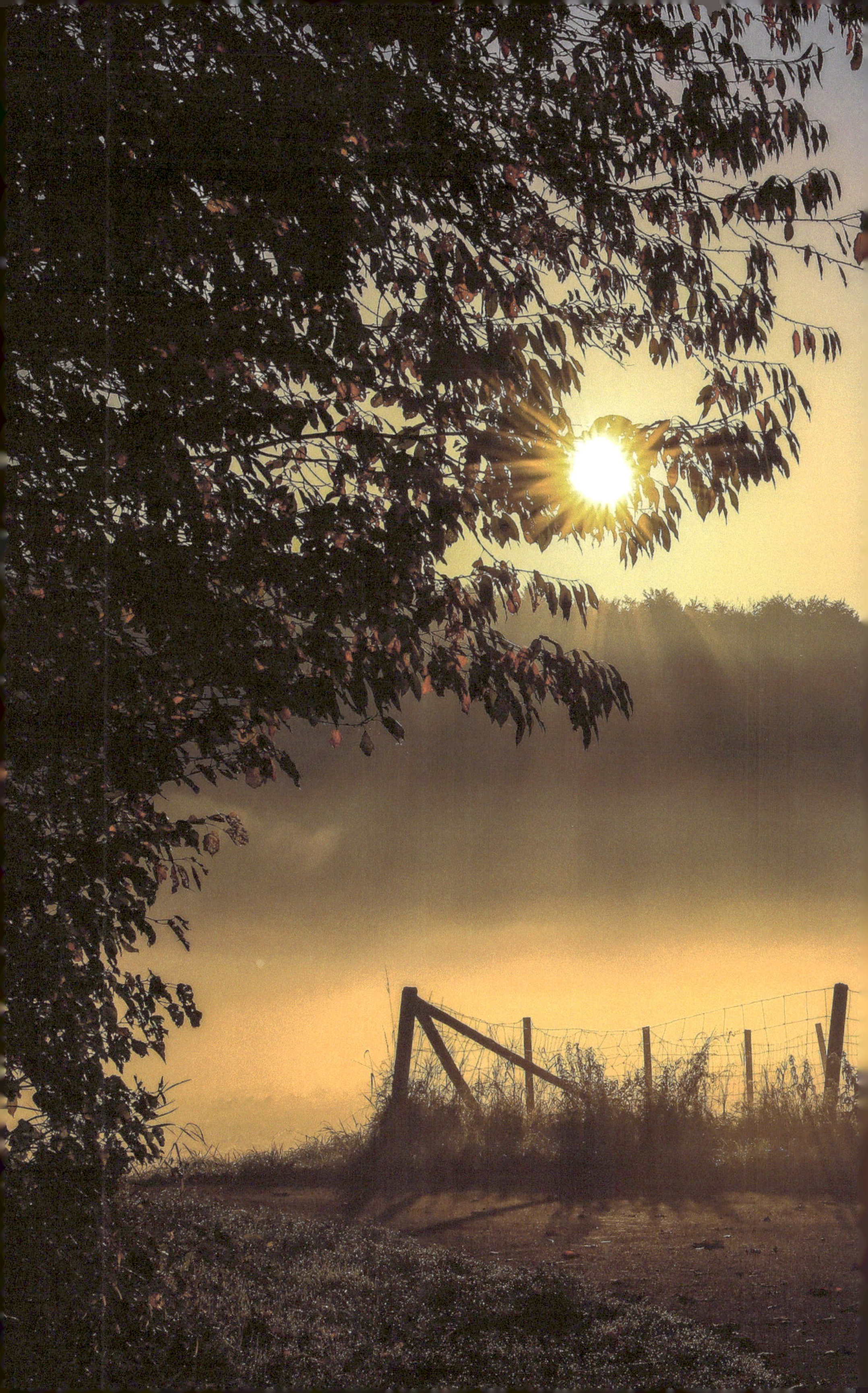

Proverbs 3-5

Trust in the Lord with all
your heart and lean not on
your own understanding.

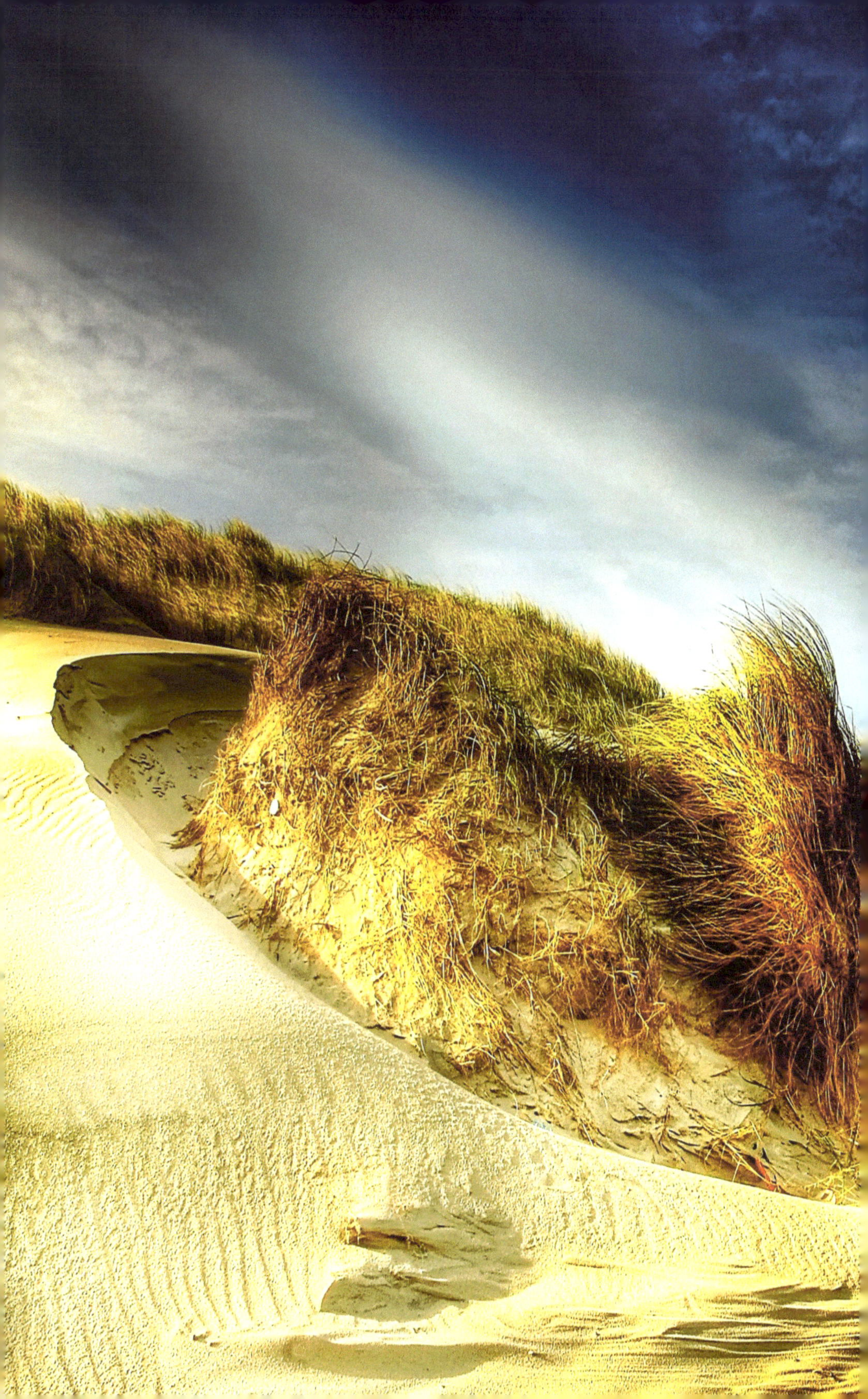

Romans 10 - 17

So faith comes from hearing, and hearing by the word of Christ.

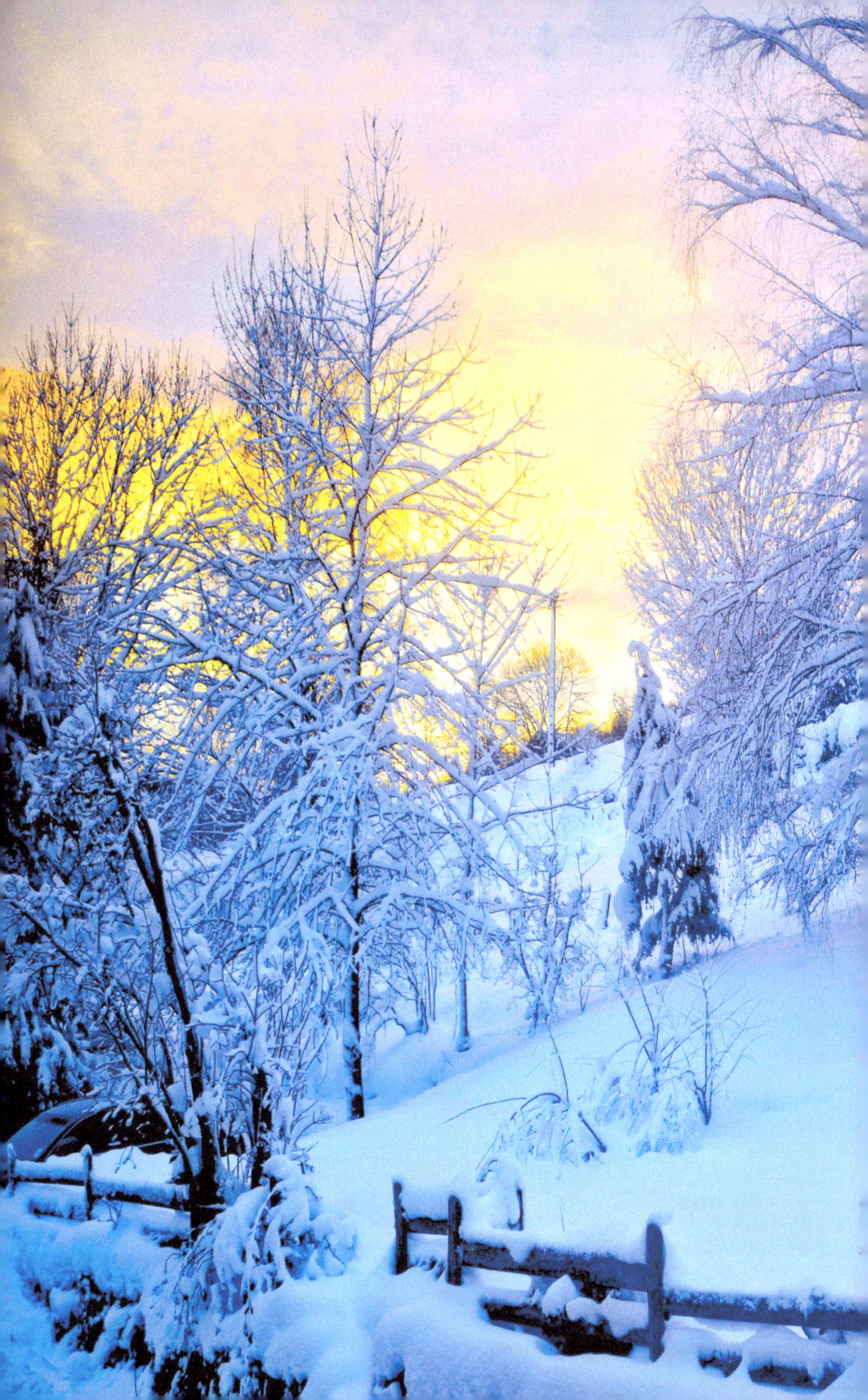

Psalms 56-11

In God I have put my
trust, I shall not be
afraid.

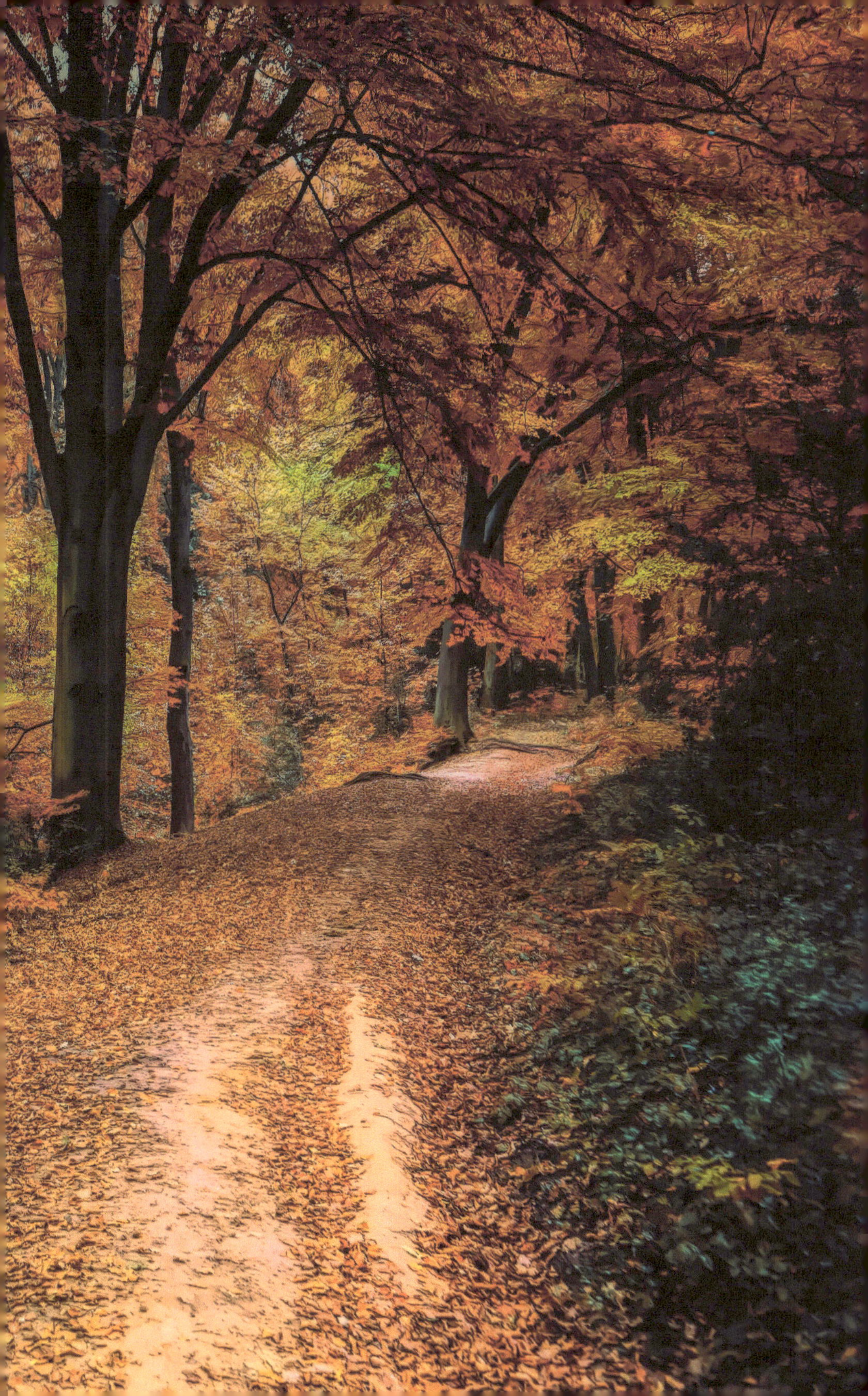

Matthew 14-31

Immediately Jesus stretched
out His hand and took
hold of him, and said to
him, "You of little faith,
why did you doubt?"

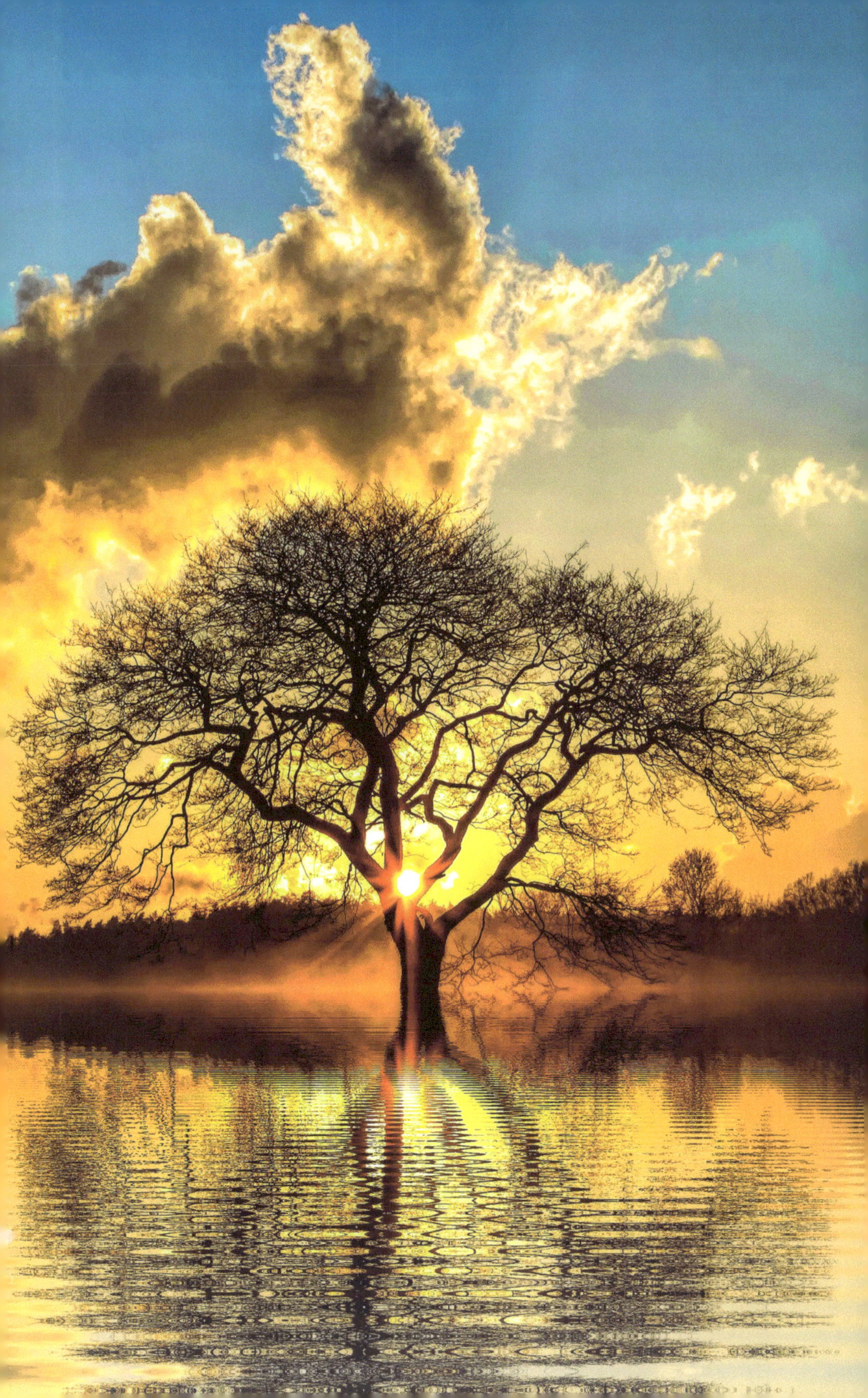

1 Corinthians 16-13

Be on guard. Stand firm in
the faith. Be courageous.
Be strong.

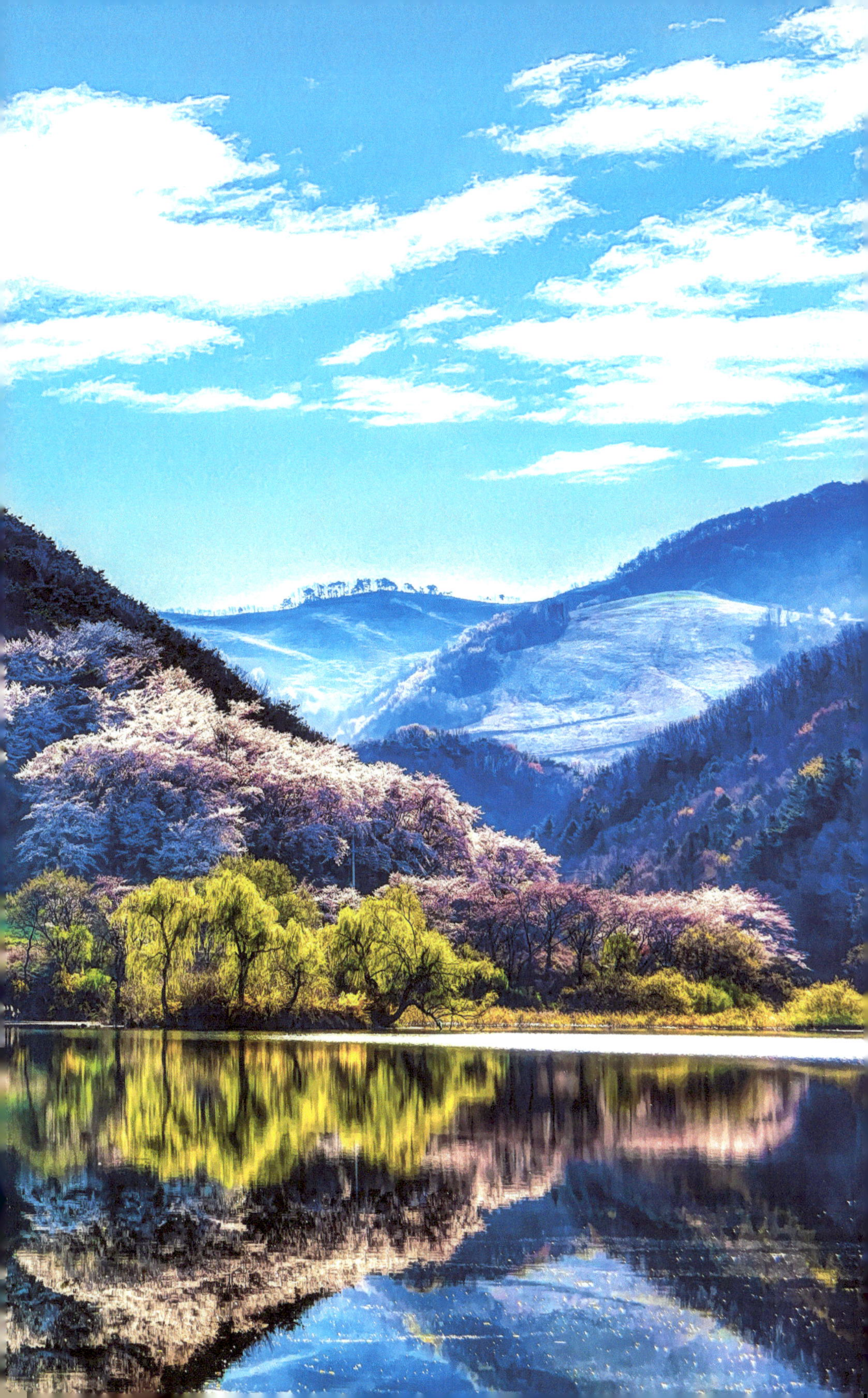

Isaiah 26-5

Trust in the Lord forever,

for in God the Lord, we have

an everlasting Rock.

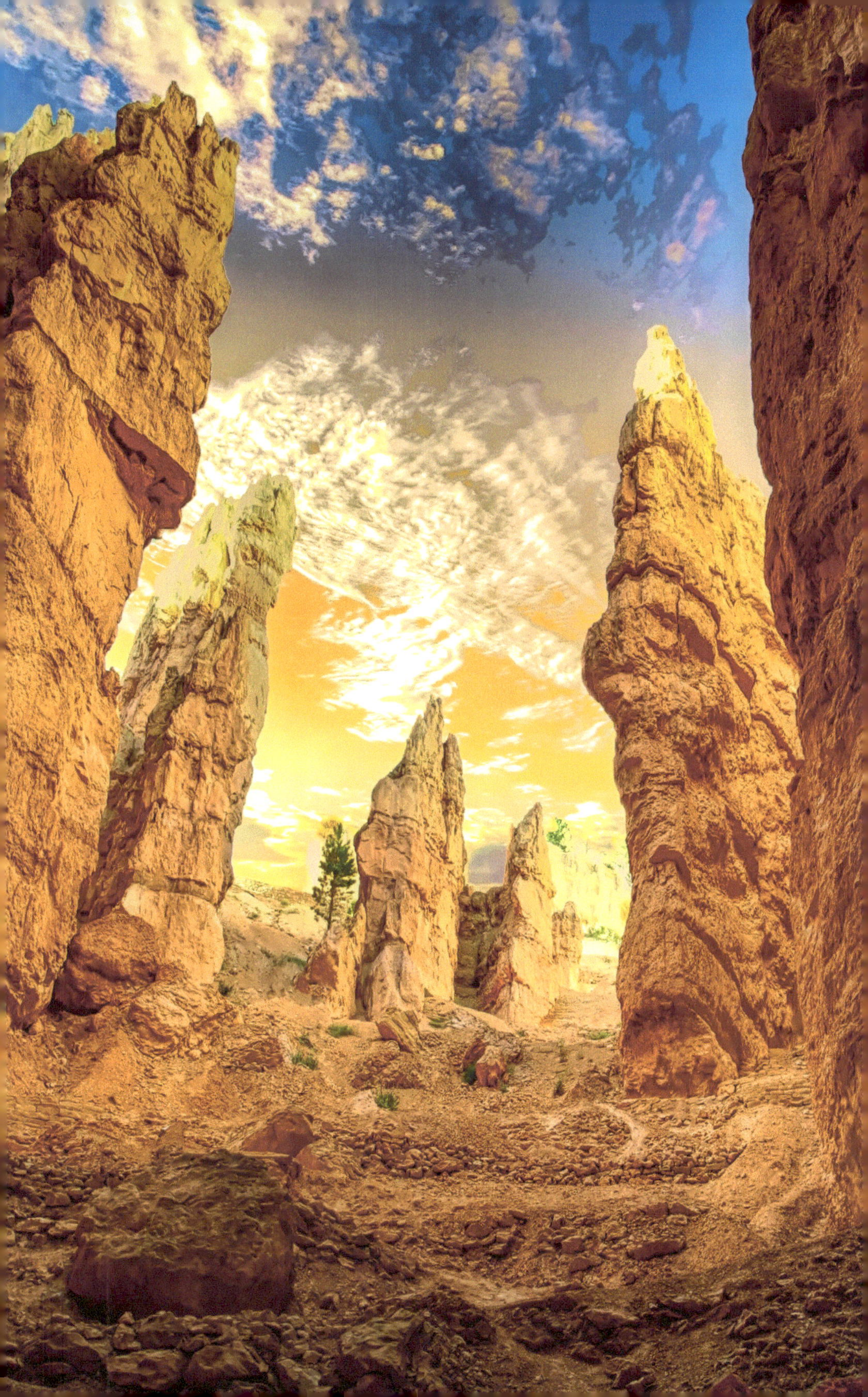

Hebrews 10-22

Let us draw near to God
with a sincere heart and
with the full assurance
that faith brings.

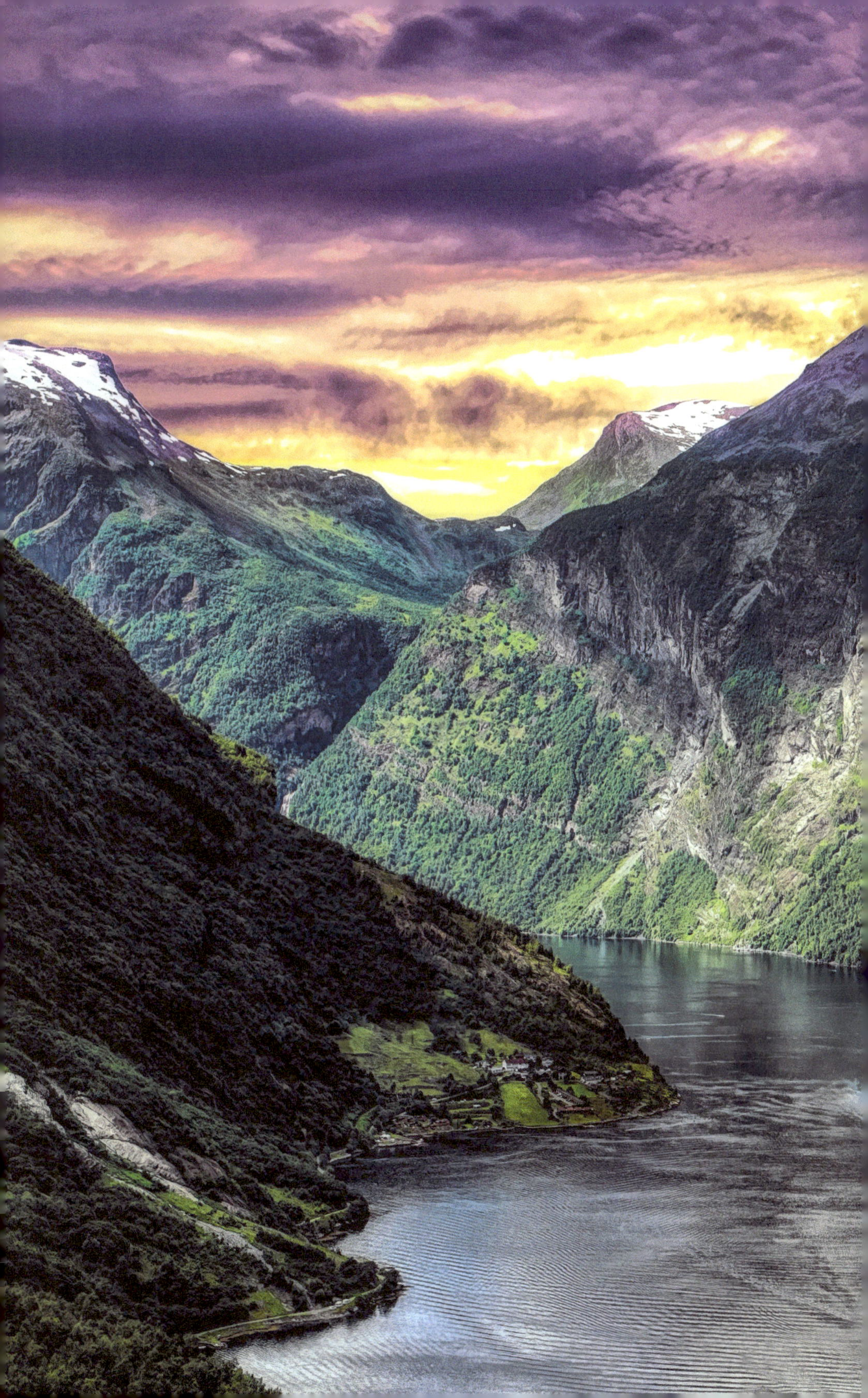

2 Corinthians 5:7

We know that while we are at home in the body we are away from the Lord, for we walk by faith, not by sight.

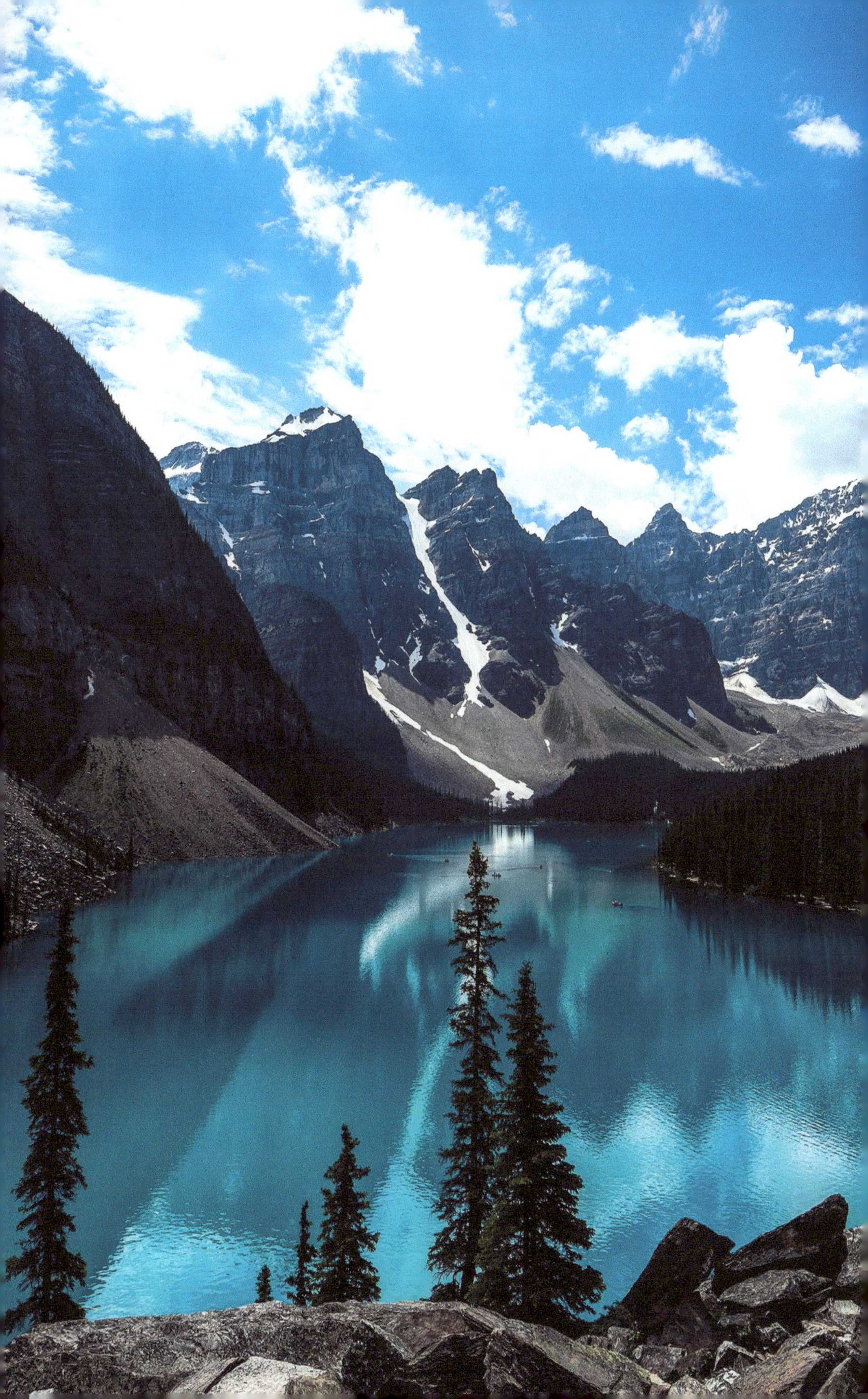

Ephesians 16-23

Peace be to the brethren,
and love with faith, from
God the Father and the
Lord Jesus Christ.

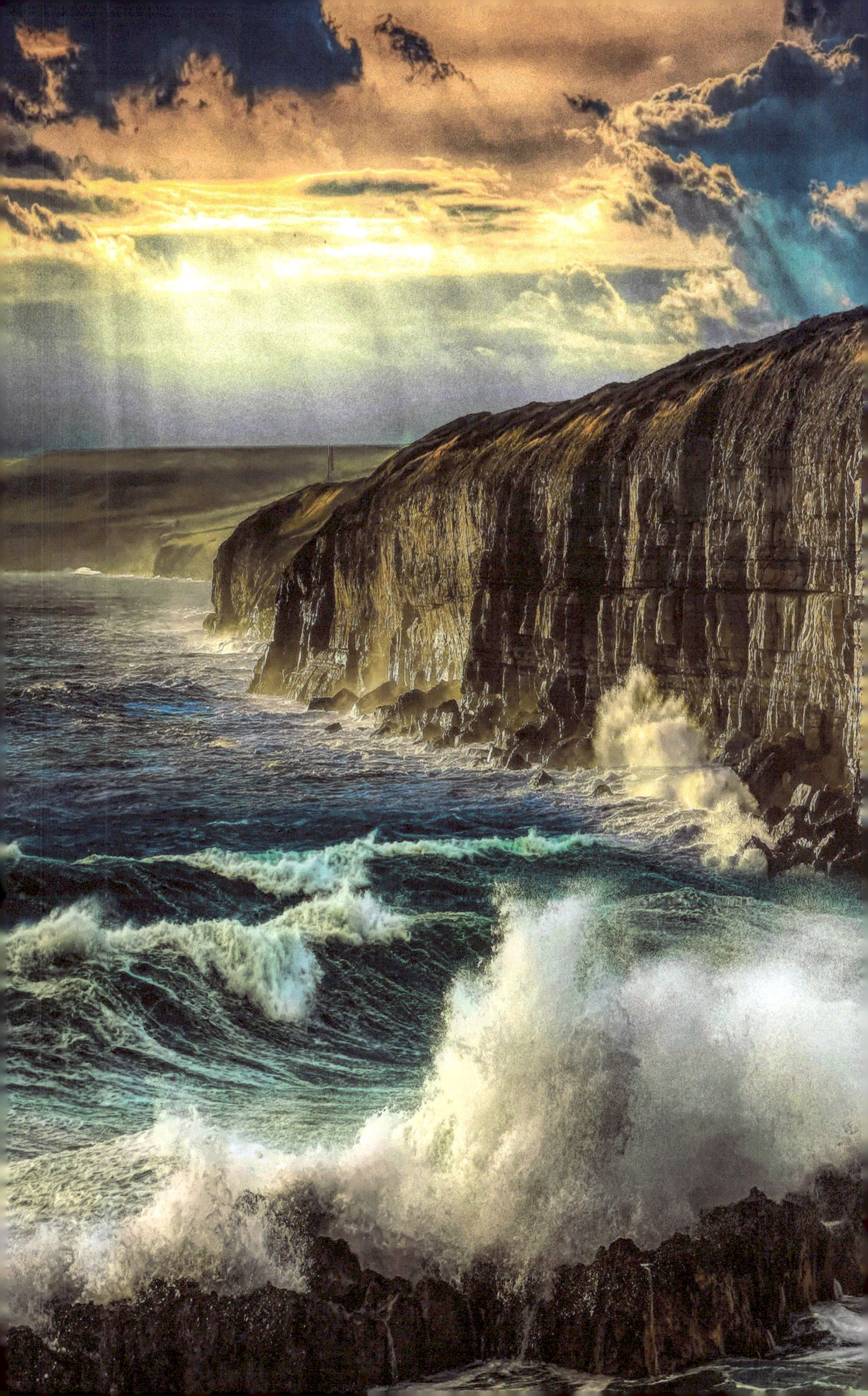

2 Chronicles 20-20

Have faith in the Lord

your God and you will

be upheld.

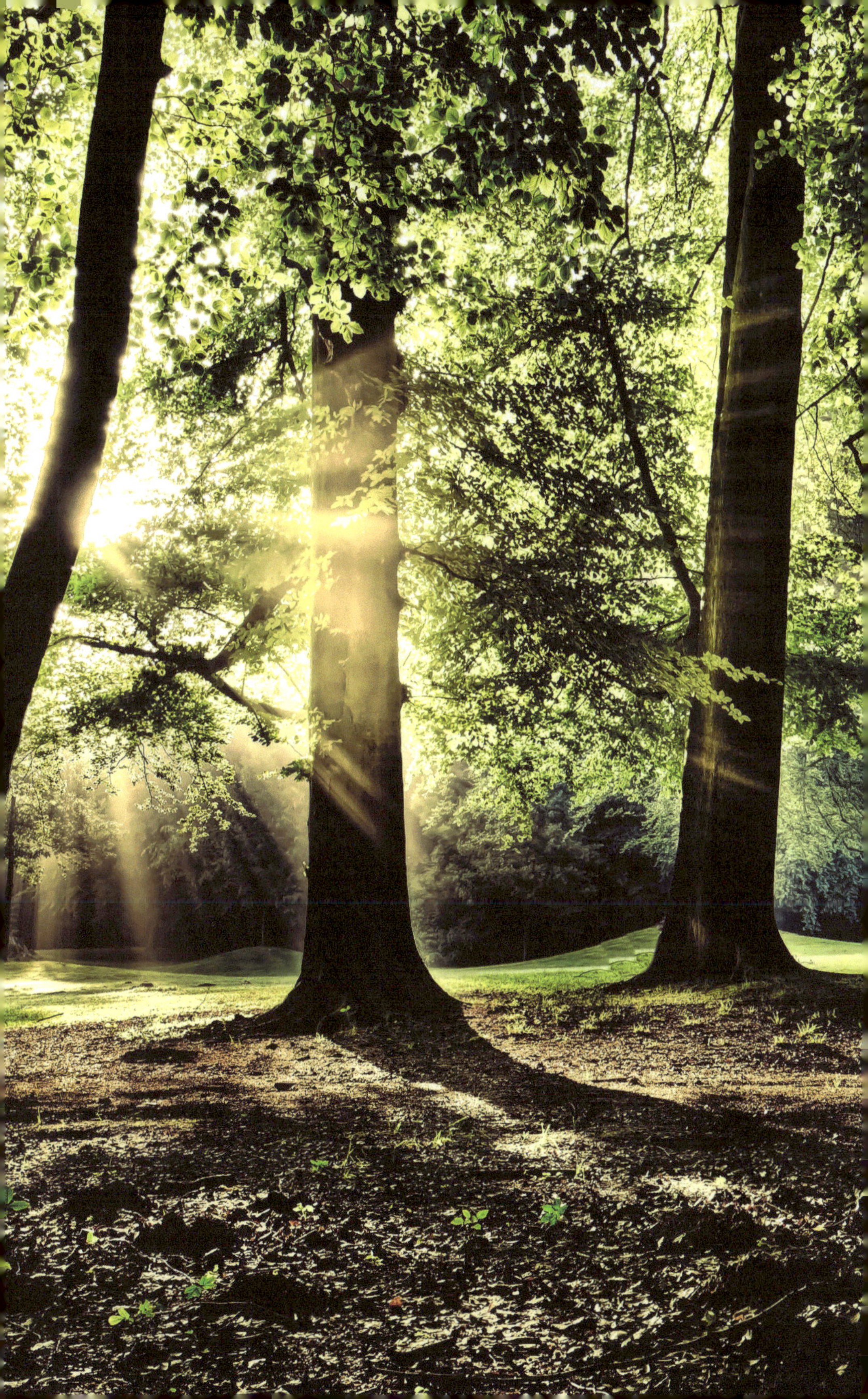

Romans 10-10

For it is with your heart that you believe and are justified, and it is with your mouth that you profess your faith and are saved.

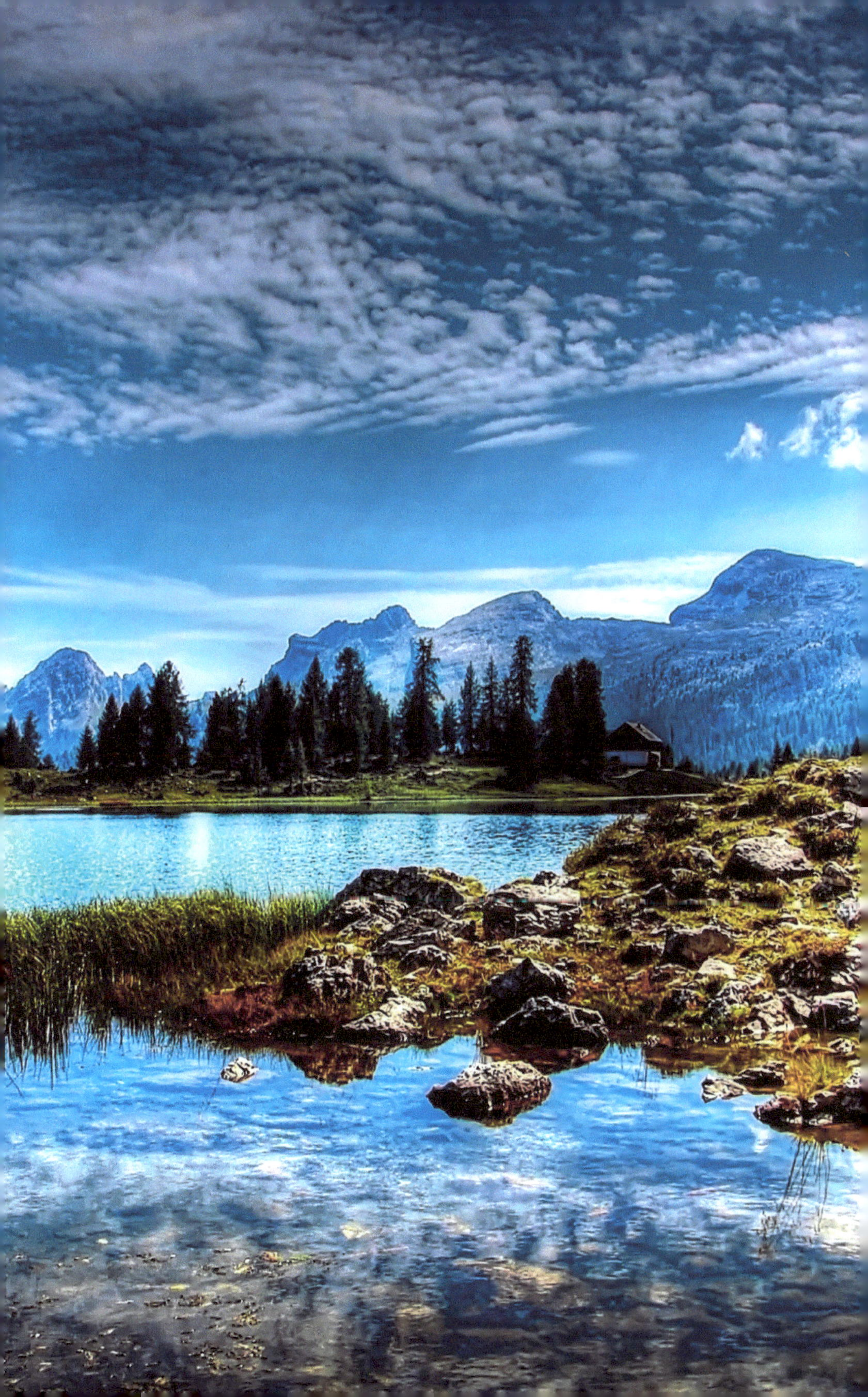

Matthew 21-22

And whatever you ask in
prayer, you will receive, if
you have faith.

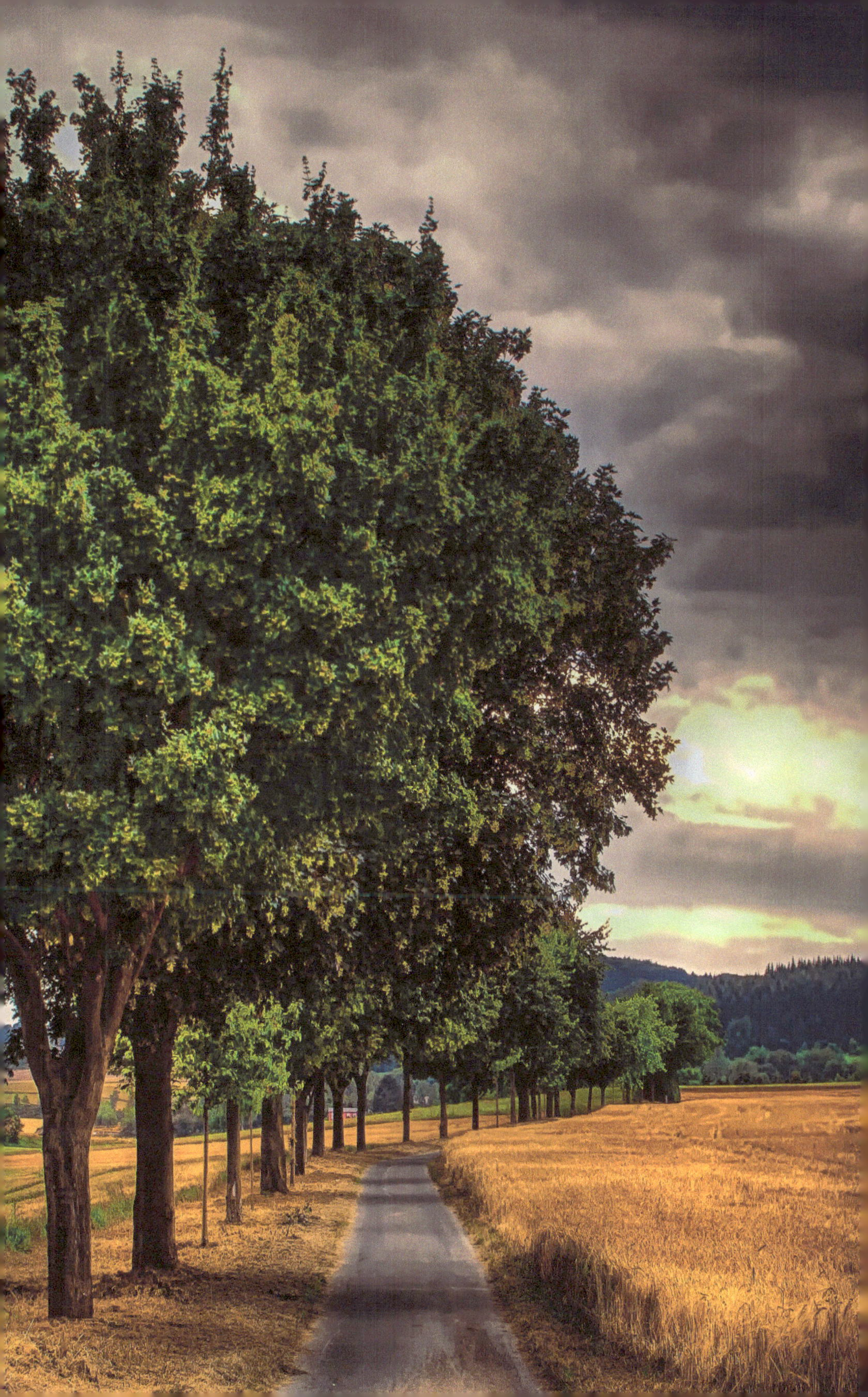

John 5-5

Who is it that overcomes
the world? Only the one
who believes that Jesus
is the Son of God.

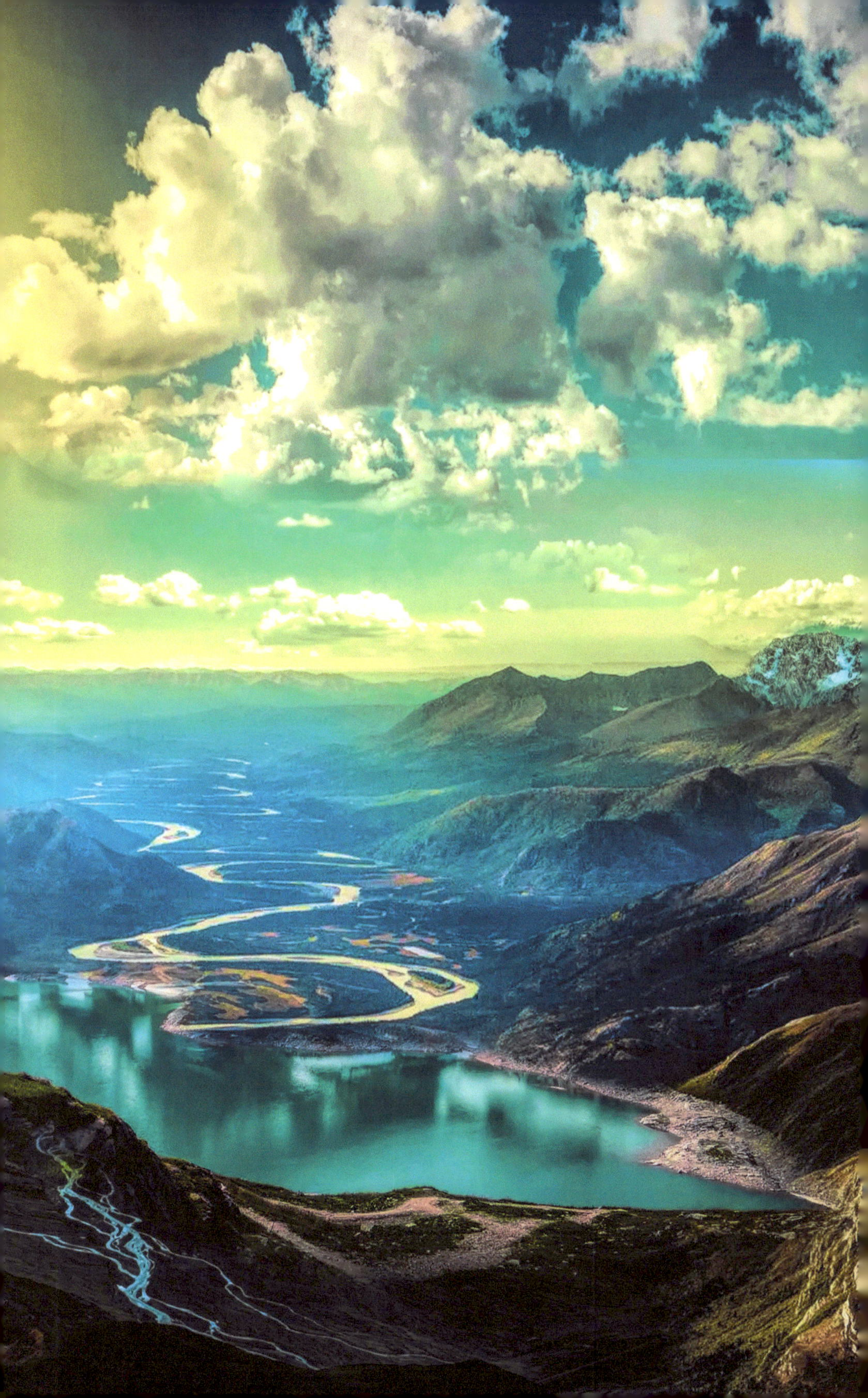

Psalms 46-10

Be still, and know that
I am God.

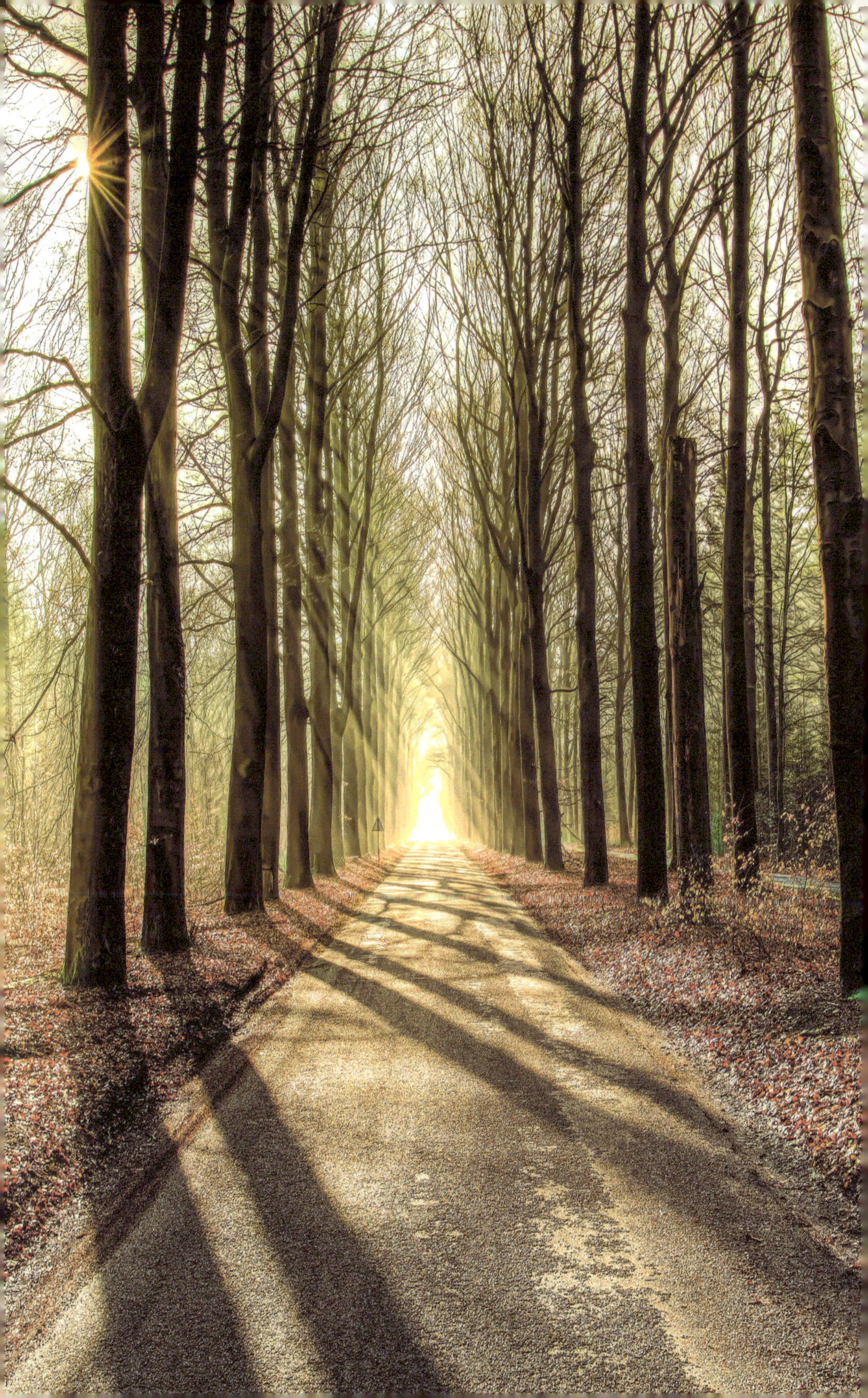

Hebrews 11-30

By faith the walls of
Jericho fell down after
they had been encircled
for seven days.

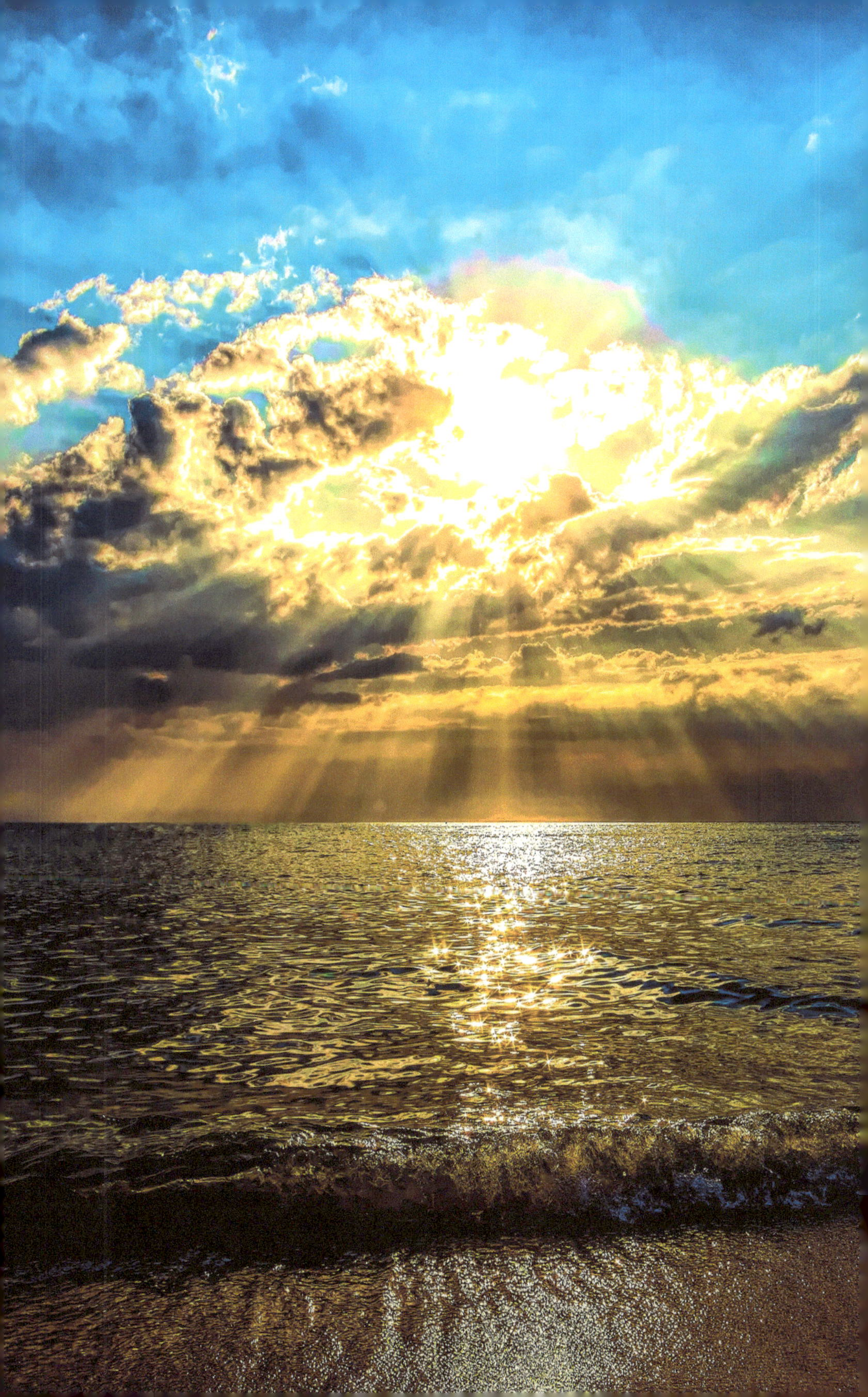